The Pi...
DOGS
IN COSTUMES

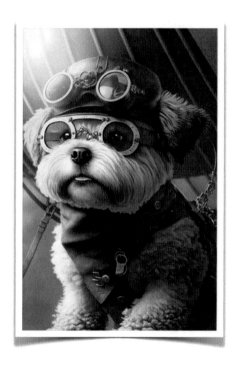

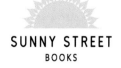

SUNNY STREET
BOOKS

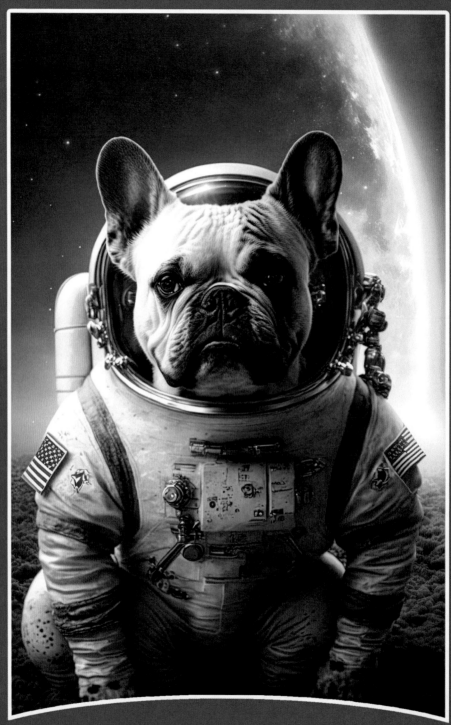

ASTRONAUT

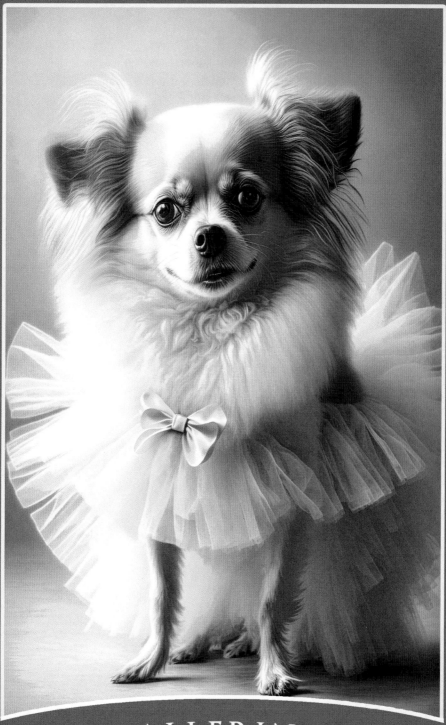

BALLERINA

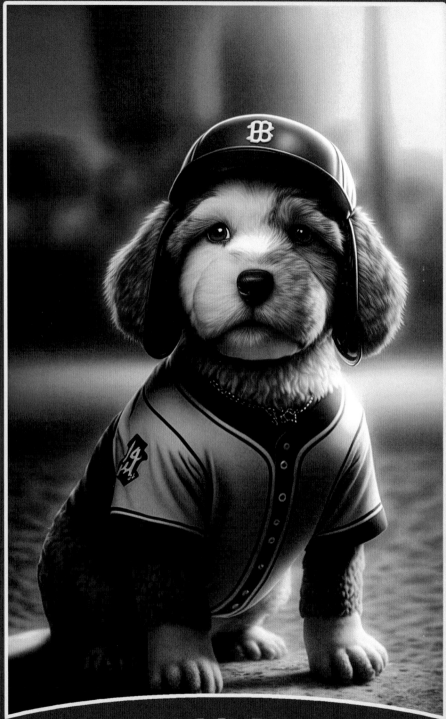

BASEBALL PLAYER

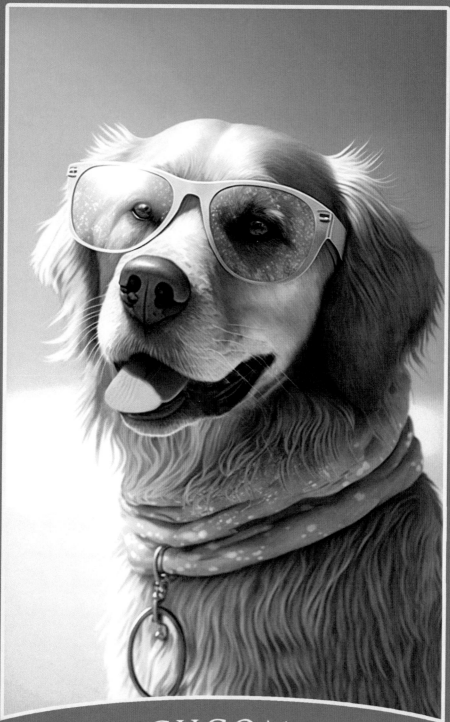

BEACHCOMBER

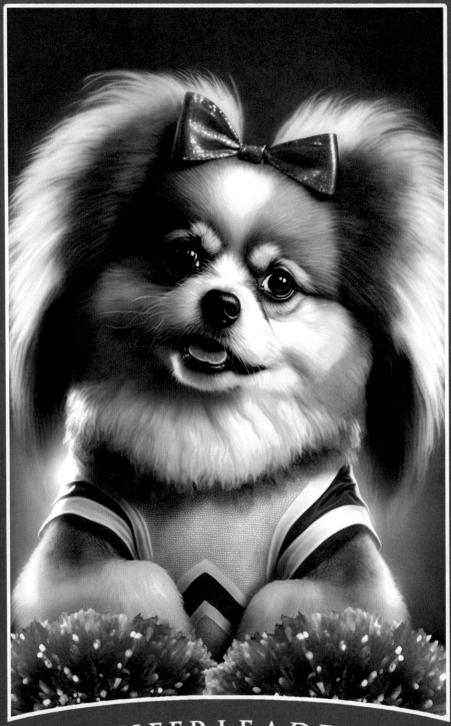

CHEERLEADER

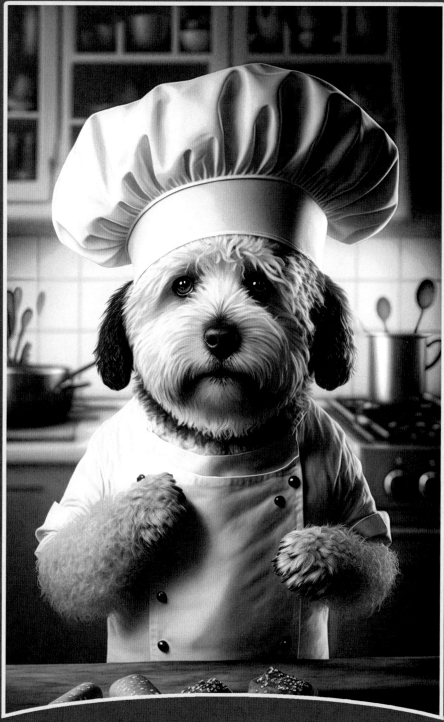

CHEF

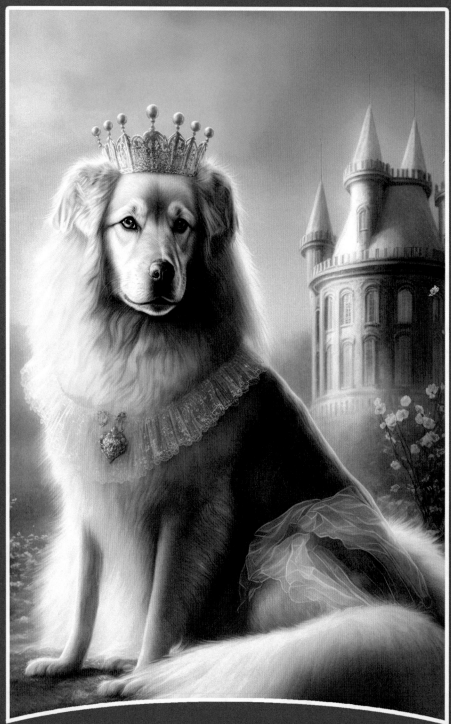

CINDERELLA

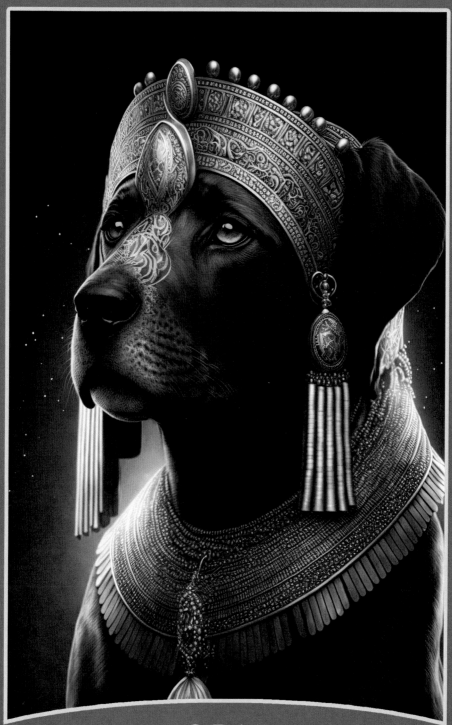

CLEOPATRA

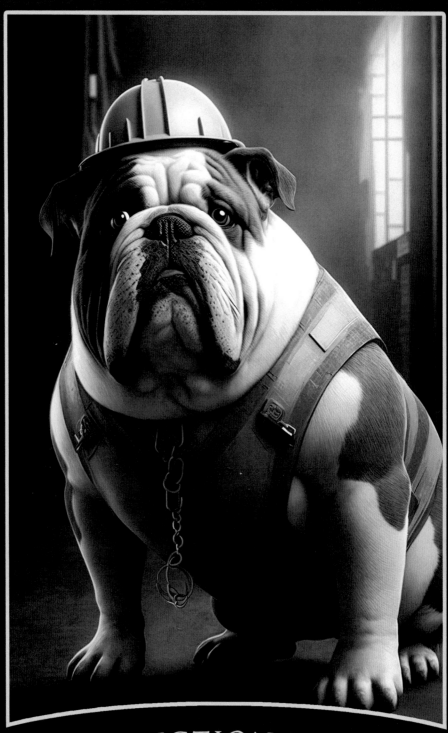

CONSTRUCTION WORKER

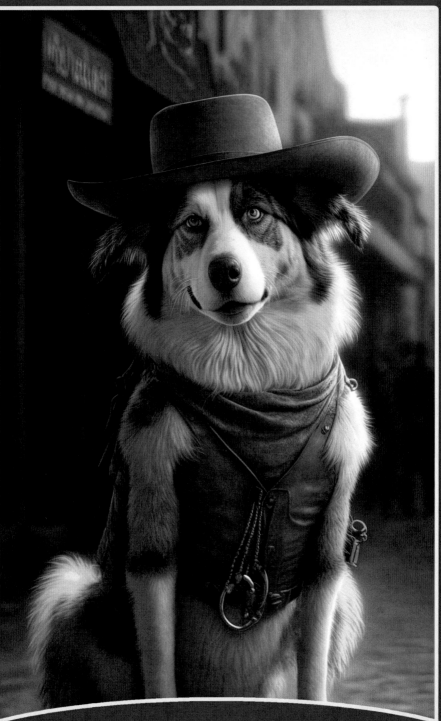

COWBOY

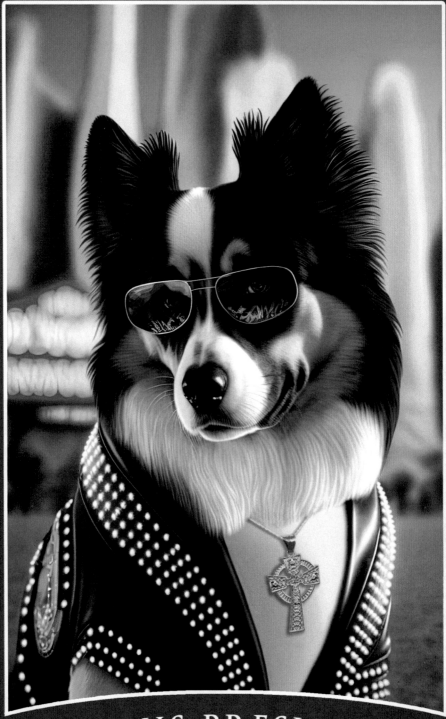

ELVIS PRESLEY

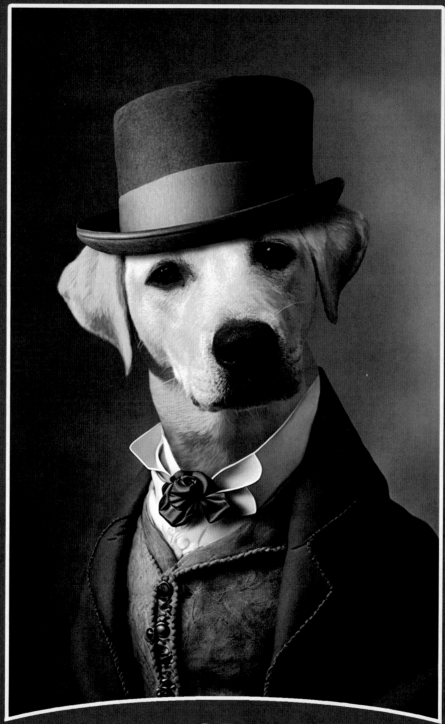

ENGLISH GENTLEMAN

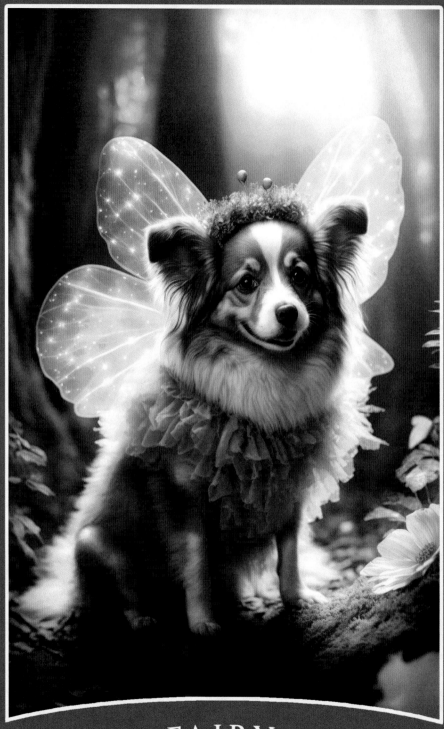

FAIRY

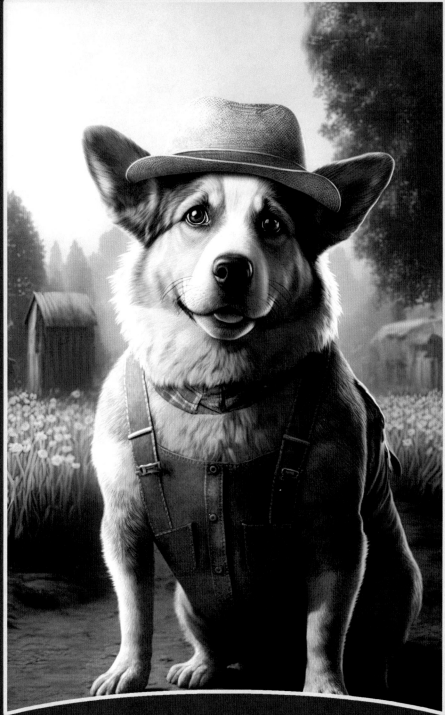

FARMER

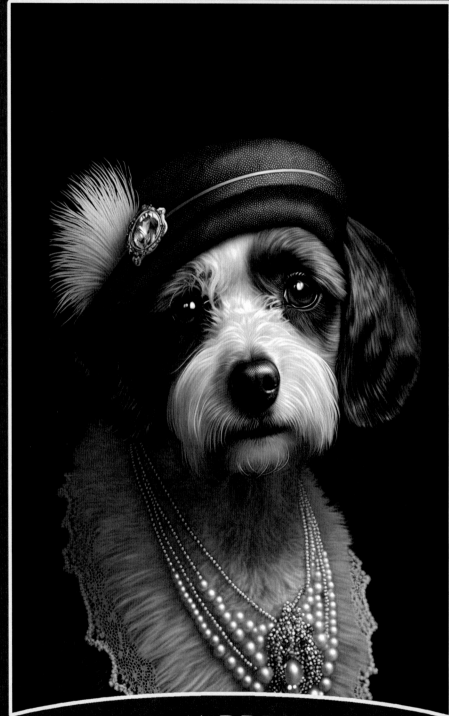

FLAPPER

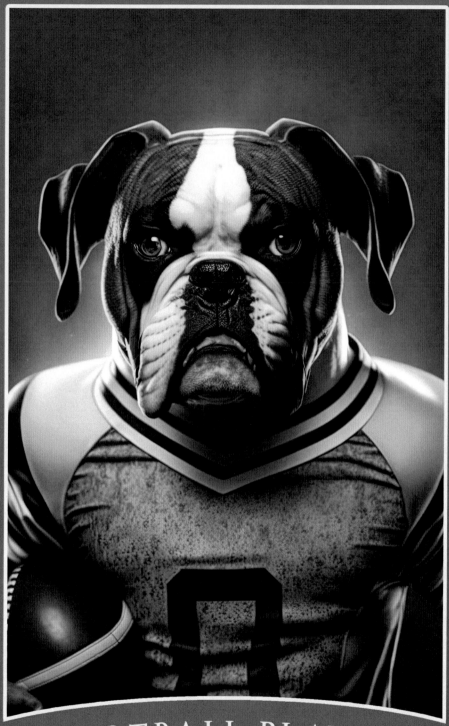

FOOTBALL PLAYER

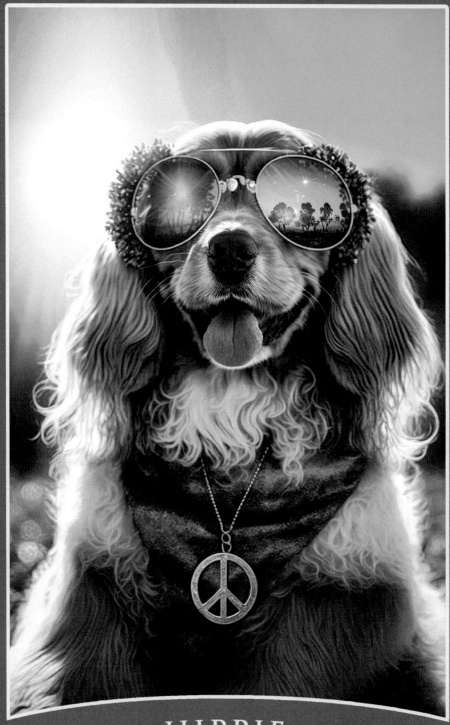

HIPPIE

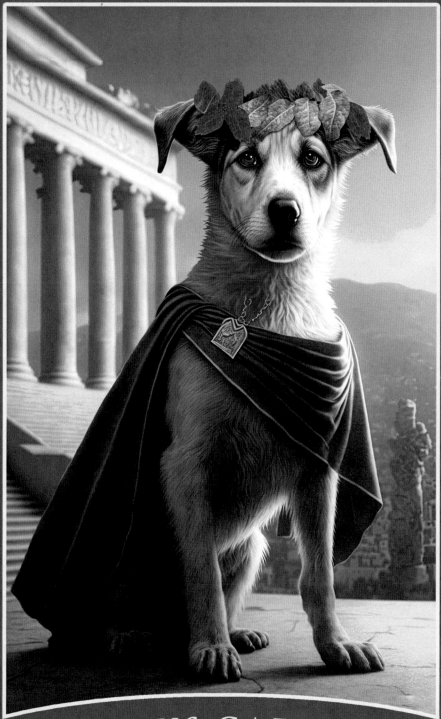

JULIUS CAESAR

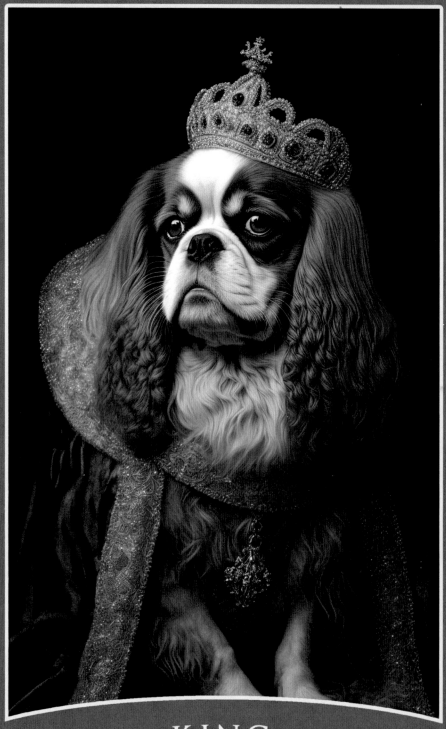

KING

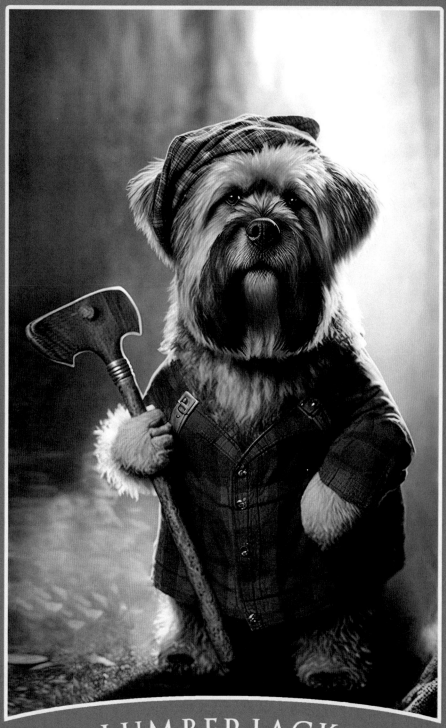

LUMBERJACK

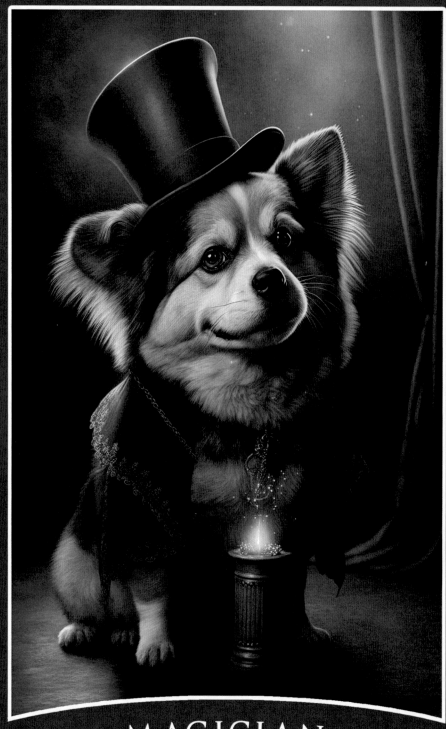

MAGICIAN

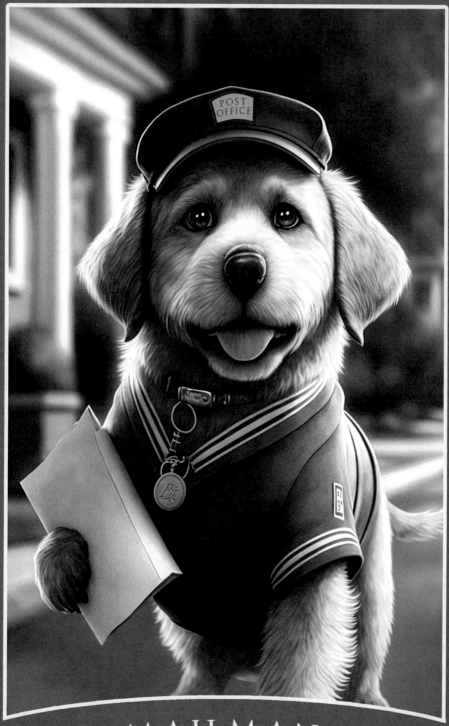

MAILMAN

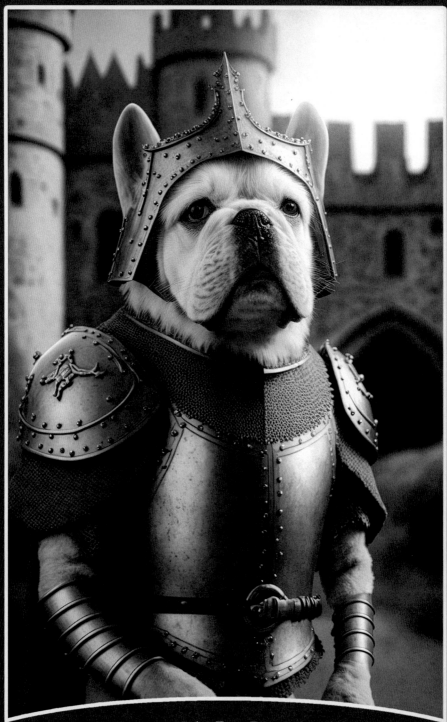

MEDIEVAL KNIGHT

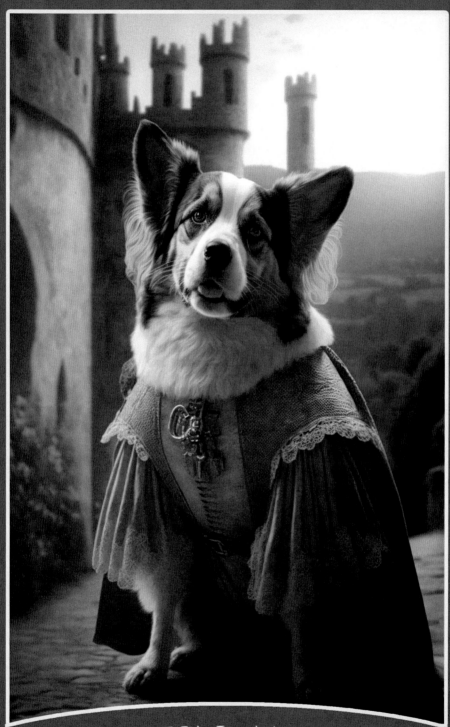

MEDIEVAL MAIDEN

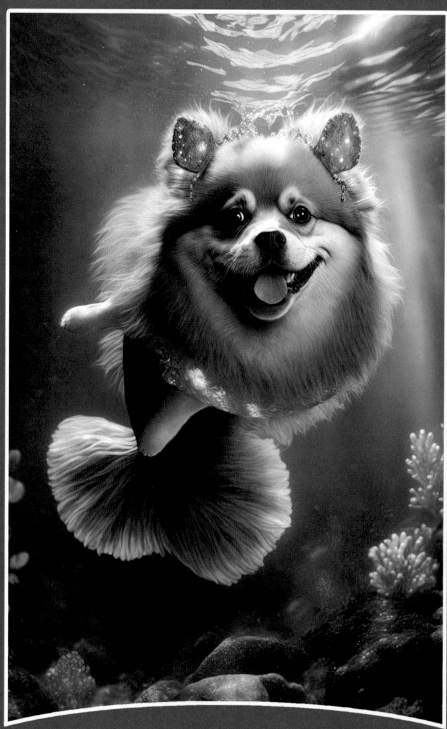

MERMAID

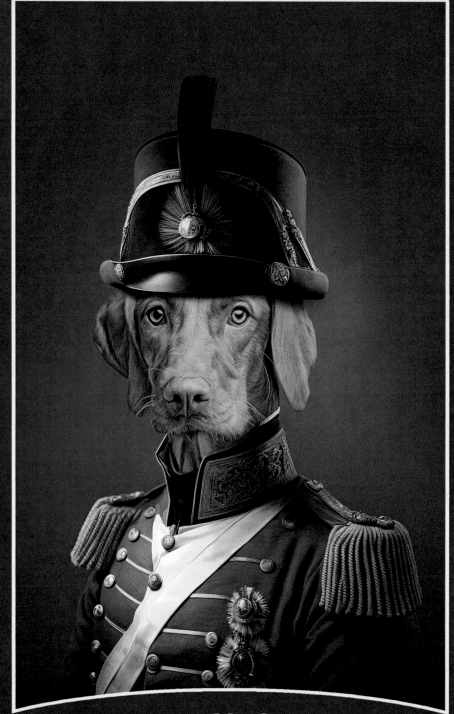

MILITARY OFFICER

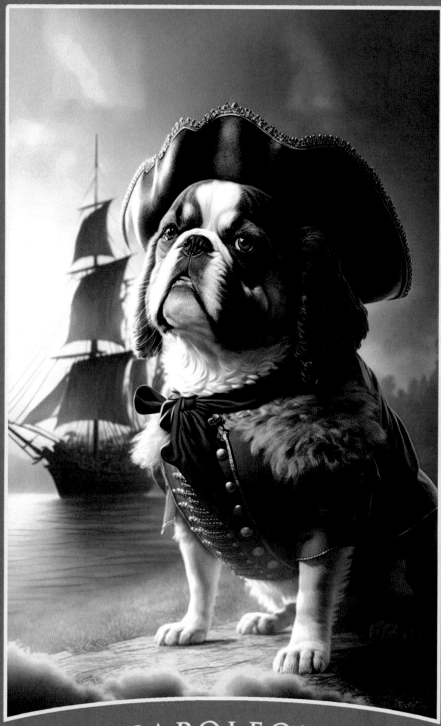

NAPOLEON

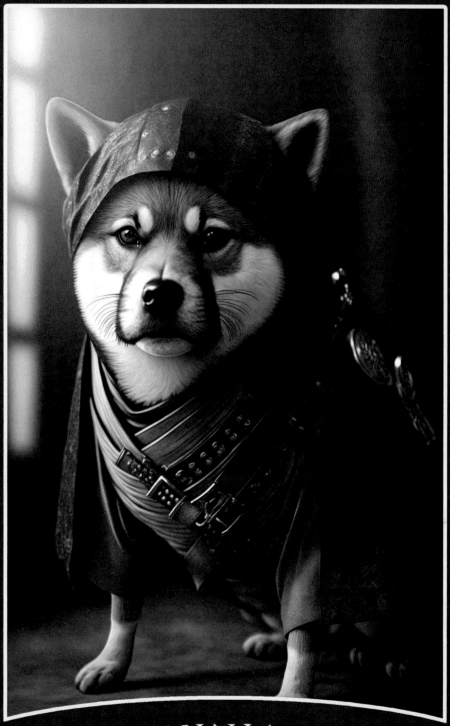

NINJA

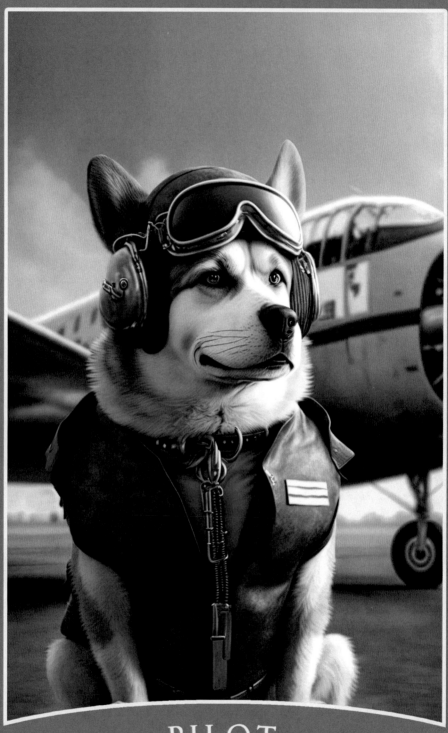

PILOT

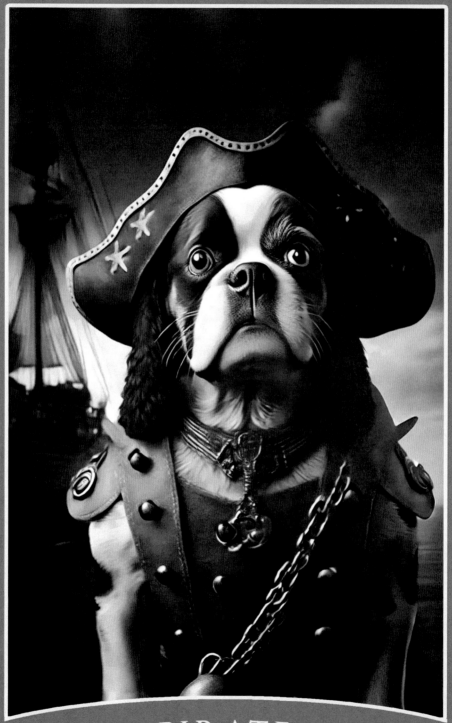

PIRATE

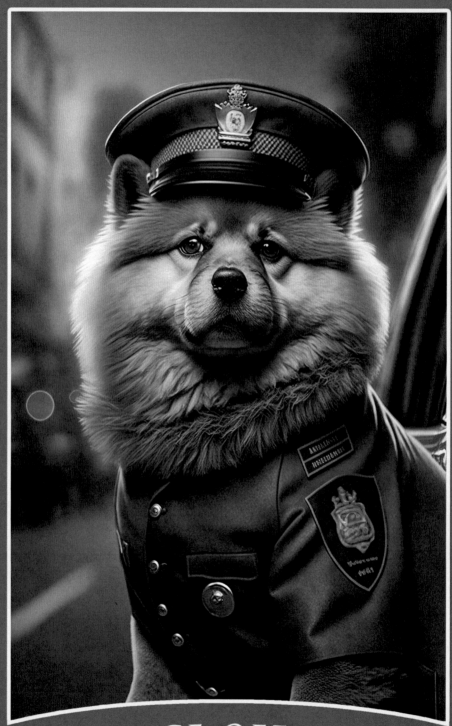

POLICE OFFICER

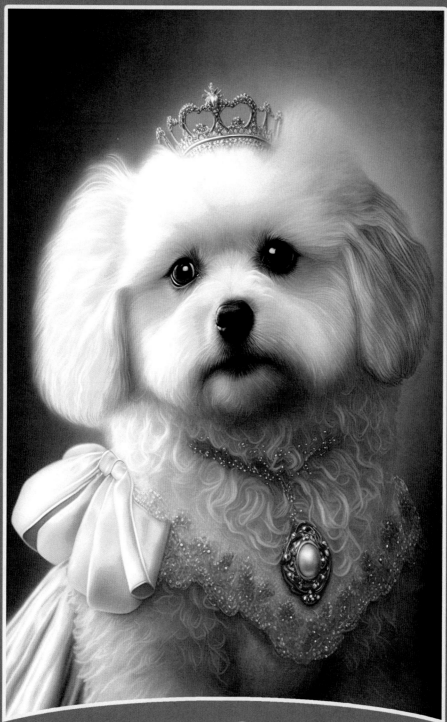

PRINCESS

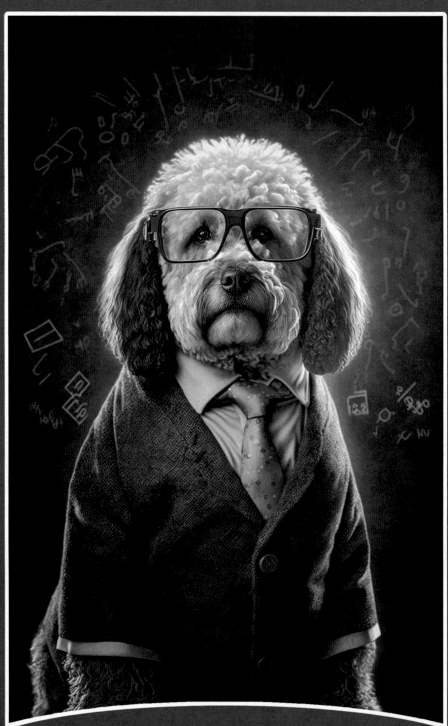

PROFESSOR

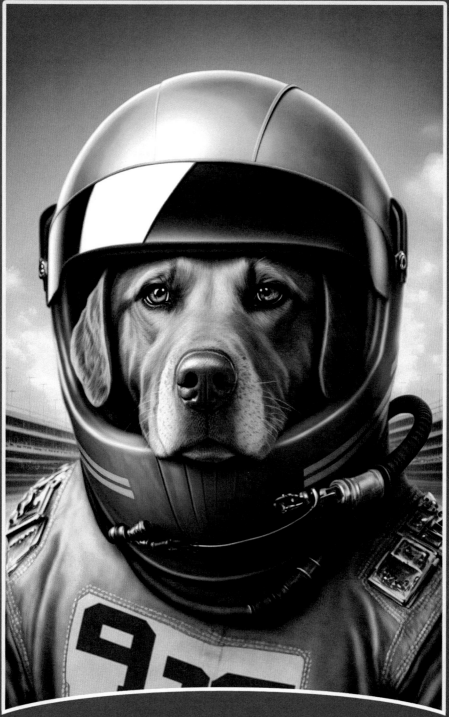

RACE CAR DRIVER

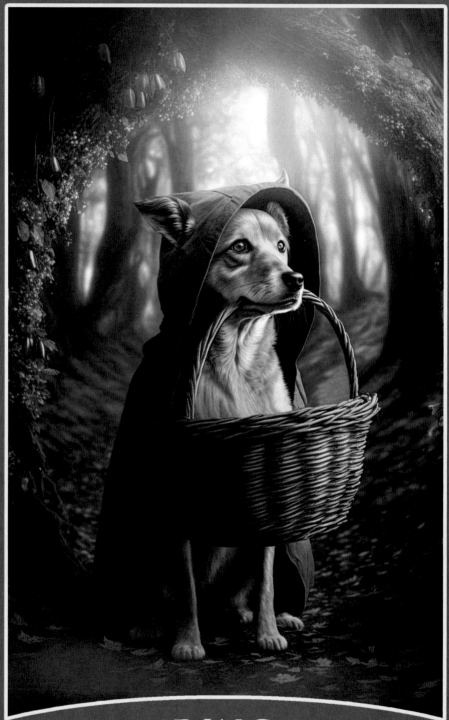

RED RIDING HOOD

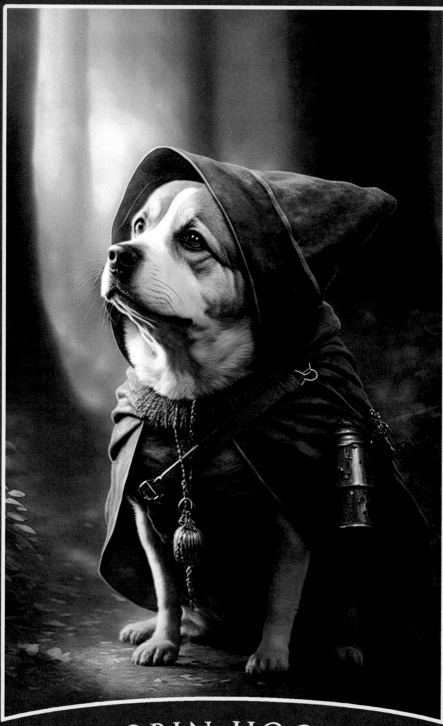

ROBIN HOOD

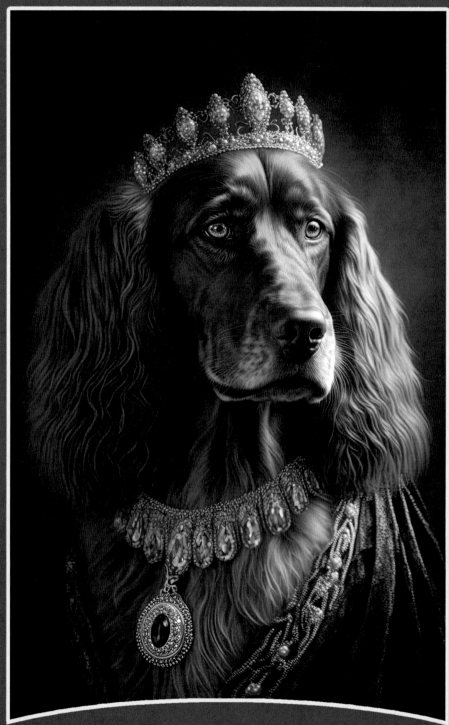

QUEEN

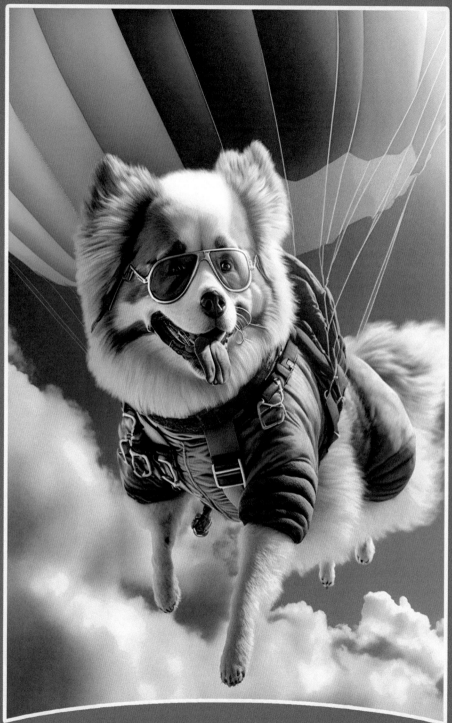

SKYDIVER

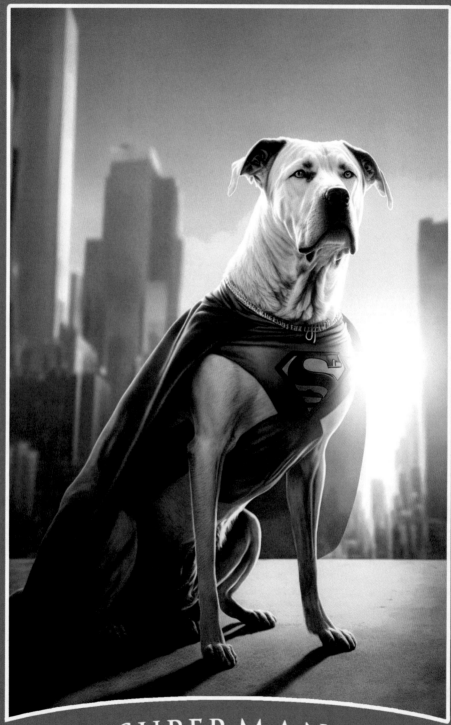

SUPERMAN

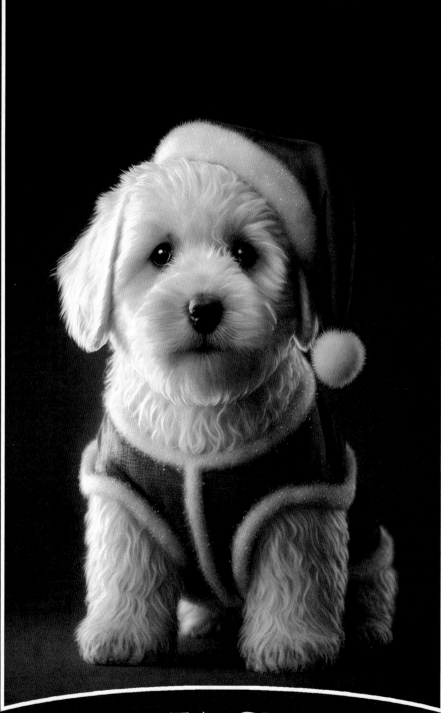

SANTA CLAUS

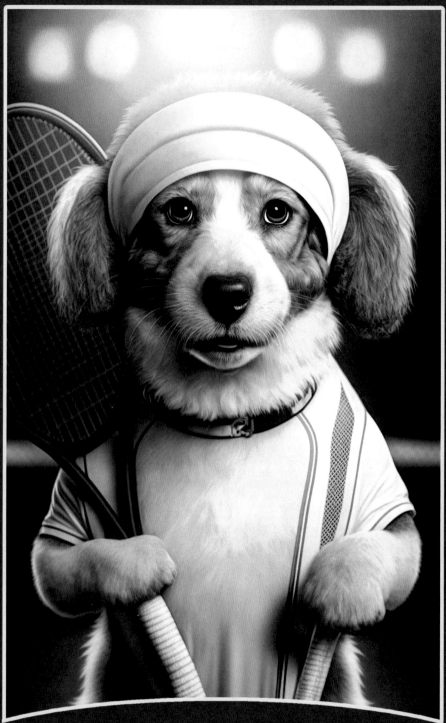

TENNIS PLAYER

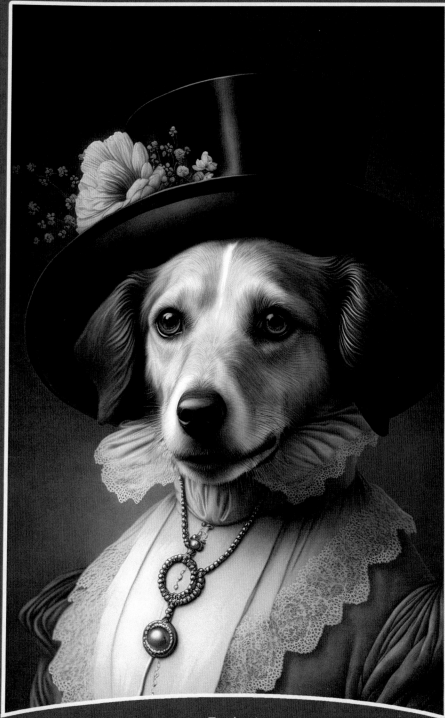

VICTORIAN LADY

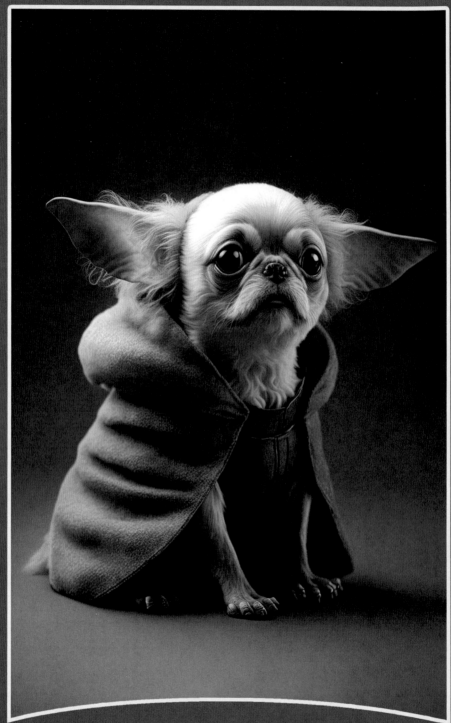

YODA